Survival Guide:

Best Ideas On How To Survive An EMP

+ 52 Effective Natural Remedies To

Survive Anywhere

Table of content:

EMP Survival Guide

**How To Survive
An Electromagnetic Pulse Attack
and Prepare Yourself For Living
After The Power Grid Goes Down**

George Robbins

EMP Survival Guide:

How To Survive An Electromagnetic Pulse Attack and Prepare Yourself For Living After The Power Grid Goes Down

Introduction: What is it? And how was it Discovered?

The acronym "EMP" stands for "electromagnetic pulse". Traces of this electromagnetic pulse were first discovered with the detonation of high yield conventional weapons. But it wasn't until the first Atomic Bomb test in July of 1945 that the effects of a large EMP burst was seriously considered. Those who worked on the Manhattan Project for the then top secret U.S. atomic weapons program were duly informed of this possibility.

Further testing of high altitude nuclear explosions in the 1950's then confirmed what researchers had long suspected all along. And it was determined that the electromagnetic pulse of a strong enough nuclear grade weapon could potentially knock out the power grid of a substantially large region, potentially even an entire nation.

But not only would an EMP knock out the standard power structure it would also fry just about any electronic device within its reach! This means that in the immediate aftermath your car wouldn't start, your cell phone won't work, and all other electronic devices and appliances in your home would be completely fried and useless. This is how a frightening new possibility of warfare known as "EMP" had been discovered.

Chapter 1: Potential Weapon Applications of EMP

As damaging as EMP weapons can be to civil infrastructure, since they are generally non-lethal in nature, their application can be very tempting to state actors. These weapons allow for a significant disruption of an enemy's capabilities without the moral baggage of being responsible for massive civilian casualties. But a truly nefarious nation could potentially use these EMP weapons in a variety of ways to *maximize casualties and destruction.* This chapter explores all of the possible applications of weapons grade EMP.

Electro Magnetic Pulse Generator

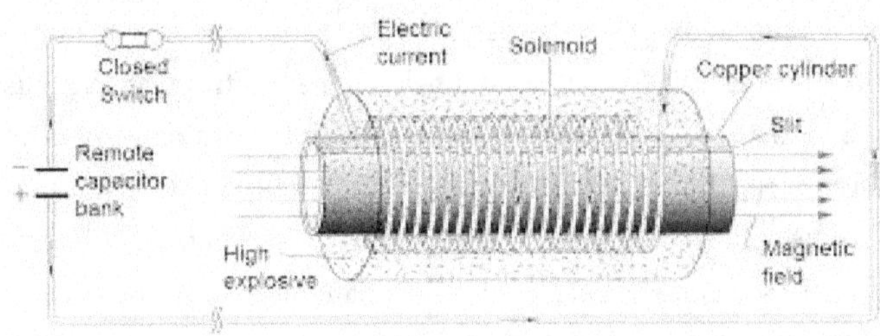

Electro magnetic pulse generators are still in development but if completed these highly focused, powerful weapons could potentially utilize microwave energy to create a massive and narrowly focused pulse that would be devastating both on the battle field and in the civilian theatre.

**Hemp**

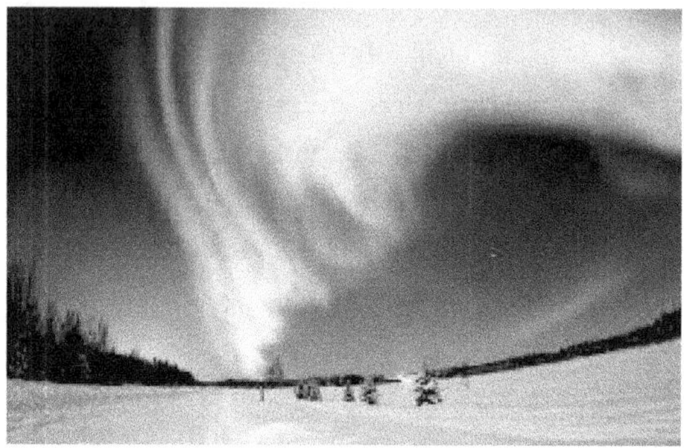

Tested with devastating success, "HEMP" refers to an instance of detonating a powerful nuclear weapon high in the atmosphere, in order to send out intense electro magnetic fields over a wide area of land below. The electromagnetic pulse created from just one instance of HEMP would be enough to fry almost all of the electronics in a large area. The wave of this pulse could potentially take out radio towers, and most power lines and cables. A HEMP weapon would also interact directly with the Earth's magnetic field, and utilize gamma rays to increase the power of the electromagnetic pulse.

Nemp

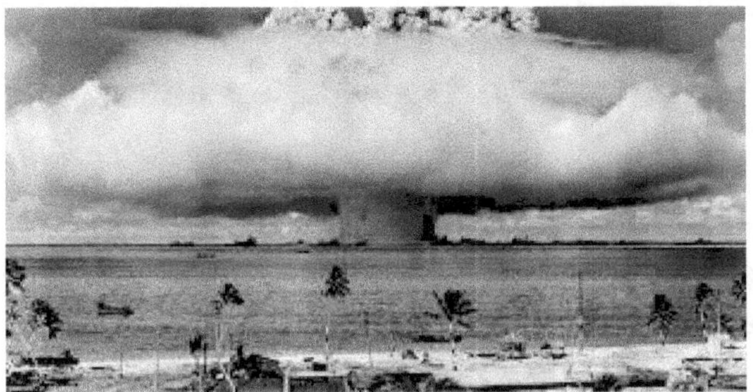

Nuclear electro magnetic pulse weapons are the standard weapons application of EMP that occurs as a direct result of a regular nuclear bomb blast. This is the general side effect of any nuclear blast but is particularly classified as such when it is intentionally use in this fashion.

<u>*E-Bombs*</u>

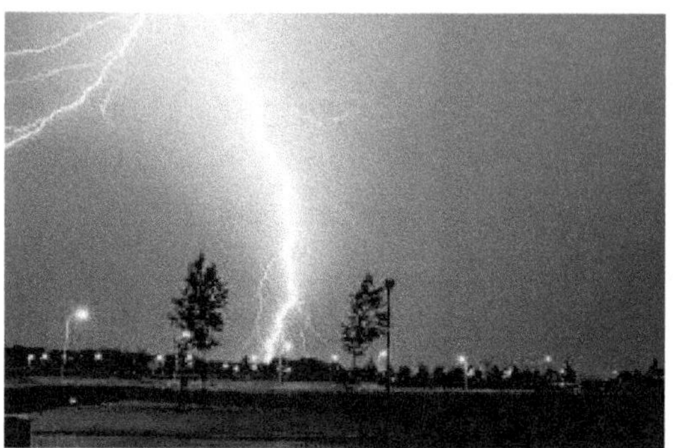

So called "E-Bombs" are highly efficient non-nuclear bombs that can unleash an intense magnetic field. These highly specialized weapons could be potentially produced so small that they could be fitted inside a suitcase. It is said that these weapons may be highly effective on the battlefield against specific military targets but would not pose that much of a threat to larger civilian infrastructure.

High Power Microwave Weapons

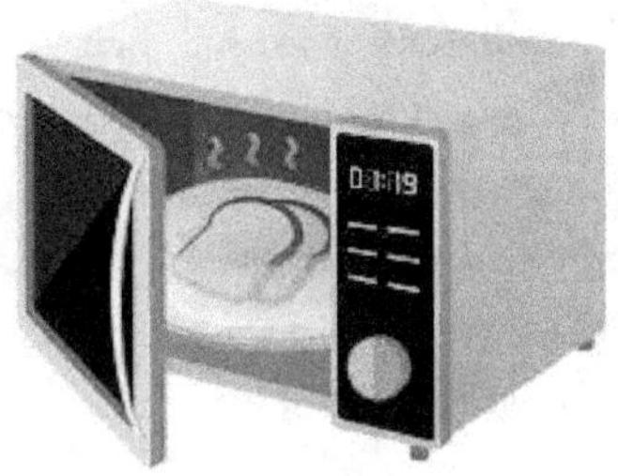

Described by the wavelength of their electromagnetic power, microwaves are used for a wide variety of applications from everything from radar to the microwave oven in your office that pops your popcorn. But HPM's or "high power microwaves" are on a whole other scale when it comes to the level of energy that is being produced.

In recent years many strides have been made to focus these HPM's into an EMP inducing weapon. By using something called a "flux compressor" these High Power Microwave Weapons can produce an incredibly formidable electromagnetic pulse that could wipe out any electrical equipment in its path. Even traditionally hardened and shielded devices are still affected by the penetrating wavelengths of High Power Microwave Weapons.

Remember when your mom told you not to stand in front of the microwave? Well there is a reason for that, because microwaves are able to permeate just about every surface, but unlike your relatively harmless microwave oven, a powerful HPM could wreak untold havoc.

Chapter 2: Ground Zero of an EMP

The ground zero of an EMP attack is certainly quite different from the ground zero of a nuclear or even conventional explosion. You won't find buildings shelled to their foundation or dead bodies smoldering in the street. The effects of an EMP are invisible and they only affect machinery, *not biological material* such as human beings consist of! In this chapter we will guide you through just what you might expect to find at the epicenter; *ground zero of an EMP attack!*

Strange Silence and Lights Out

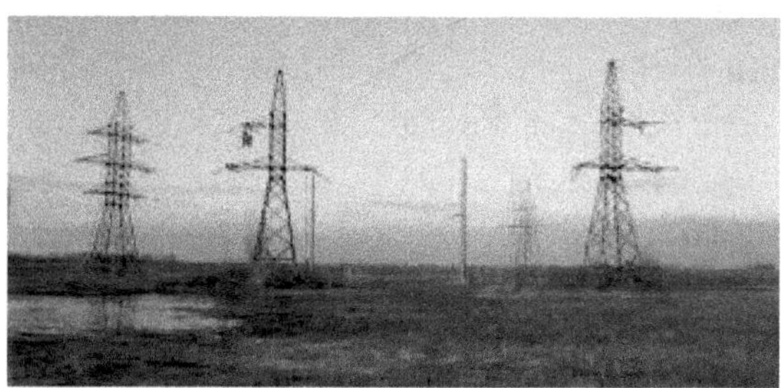

The calm quiet of the aftermath of an EMP burst is one of the first standout features of such an attack. Imagine sitting down in your living room during a typical afternoon with TV blaring the news, dishwasher whirring through the latest round of dishes, your kids blaring music down the hall, and your next door neighbor cutting grass with the roar of a lawn mower. But in a split second, suddenly everything stops, no more TV, no more dishwasher, no more music, and even the lawnmower; inexplicably go quiet.

At first you think there must have been a local power outage; a simple enough explanation right? You instinctively reach for your phone to dial up your local power company, but you find the screen blank and lifeless.

You stare in disbelief thinking, "Didn't I just charge my phone? What is going on here?" Unable to call out for help you decide to take a step outdoors. But as you step outside and greet your neighbor whose *gas powered* lawn mower strangely conked out right when your power went out, the two of you turn to see another neighbor's car slowly skidding to a halt at the end of the street.

Another odd coincidence but you shrug it off as inopportune car trouble. You then see another neighbor futilely attempting to start his own car, putting in his key and cranking the ignition, but nothing but silence. Soon enough you would find that this silence in the aftermath of an EMP attack is permeating your entire neighborhood and the entirety of the ground zero of the electro magnetic pulse that has been unleashed. If the EMP burst occurred in the middle of the night the effect would be even more dramatic because all of your lighting would go out.

Even more disturbing, you would find that the trusty flashlight app on your phone is useless because all of your cell phones are fried! And even if you manage to fish out an old fashioned standalone "flashlight" (remember those?), you would be greatly distressed to find that even this simple instrument of illumination wouldn't work either! Your classic flashlight and the additional pair of batteries you stashed away, would be completely useless.

This is just how pervasive the electromagnetic pulse is, although you as a biological human being do not feel the pulse, in a split second it has flashed through every single piece of equipment you own. Sitting in the dark, you and your family will quickly realize that the only source of lighting available to you would be an old fashioned candle. In the aftermath of an EMP many will be wandering through their blackened neighborhoods with makeshift lanterns looking like they came straight out of the 1800's. This is the strange new world that is the ground zero of an EMP.

Spoiled Food

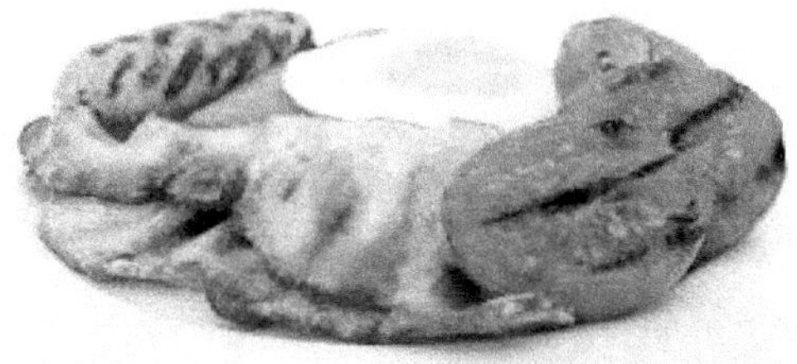

Besides the loss of our electronic devices, communication, and being able to travel freely down the road, the next biggest struggle will come from our refrigerator. Being left without power for days on end will obviously cause a massive spoilage of food. Knowing as much—in the immediate aftermath of an EMP attack—you should rank all of your food from the "most perishable" to the "least perishable".

You should then make it a priority to eat the most perishable items first. This means that for all of your food that you know will not last more than a couple of days unrefrigerated, you should eat as much of it as possible, you could even be a bit altruistic and share some of your food with your neighbors.

It's going to go bad anyway so you might as well create some good rapport with your neighbors. The least perishable food such as crackers, canned goods, and dried pasta, should be saved for the long haul, since this is food that you can rely upon in the intervening weeks without fear of it spoiling.

<u>***Distress in the Hospital***</u>

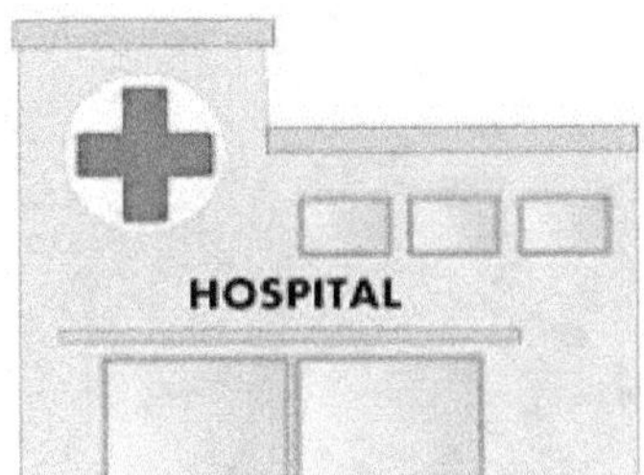

Even though an EMP blast would not directly kill anyone on the ground, the after affects could lead to significant casualties. And the most vulnerable of our population—those being cared for in our hospitals—would face the most dire of consequences. If an EMP successfully knocks out all power to the local grids, even generators wouldn't work and hospitals would truly be in the dark.

Patients in critical condition hooked up to life support would be the first to perish, flat lining as the machines that help keep them breathing go offline. After these patients perish, the next in line are those that are not necessarily hooked up to life support apparatus but who need certain life giving therapies and treatments that the power blackout would deprive them of.

After a few days these patients would die as well. One of the most disturbing aspects of an EMP is the high level of dead that it would leave in one of the most vulnerable segments of our population; those suffering from medical conditions. As you can see, such a dastardly attack would indeed bring about massive incidents of distress in our hospital system.

Social Chaos

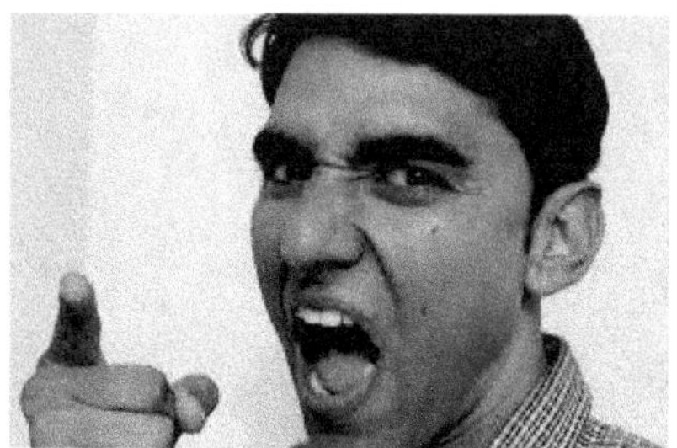

Complete social breakdown would be the biggest fear of those trying to keep the peace in the aftermath of an EMP. With food spoiled, neighborhoods completely blacked out, and with no transportation to flee, citizens will feel cornered, and the propensity of civil unrest will be extraordinarily great.

How do you control a population that is on the brink of starvation, suffering a wide variety of medical illnesses, and with no solution in sight have lost all faith in government? It would be a difficult task for any leader to rein in such social chaos. And in such a tragic situation, a nation's own members could become the greatest threat of them all.

Chapter 3: Is EMP a Real Threat? And By Whom?

North Korea has been threatening to "incinerate" the United States for several years now. And now that the U.S. has a President that seems to fight fire *with fire*, even going so far as to state to the United Nations that if the U.S. is provoked, North Korea will be "destroyed", the threat from N.K. seems to loom largest. But North Korea is certainly not the only country that could surprise Western Civilization by turning the lights off with an EMP blast. There are several actors that could carry out such an attack. In this chapter we will outline some of the more plausible of these nightmare scenarios.

Surprise Attack by Russia

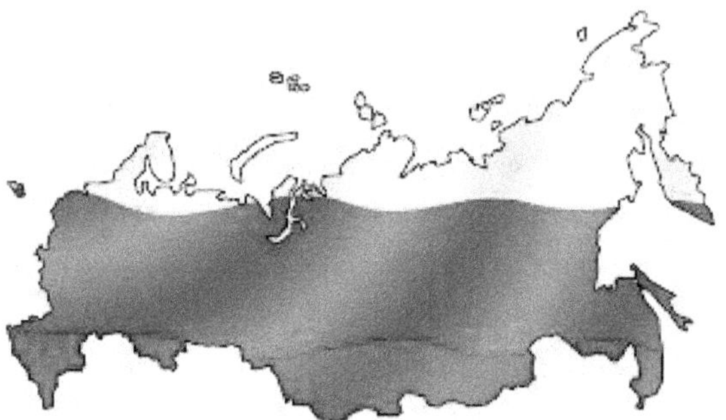

Many have joked and poked fun at those who bring up any concern in regard to tensions between the United States and the former Soviet Union. But although the Cold War is long over, and we live in a very different world, the fact still remains that the United States and Russia are the two most powerful militaries on the planet and even if these two nations are the best of friends today (contrary to what most policy wonks believe) it wouldn't take much for this relationship to deteriorate.

And having that said, Russia—of all nations—is rumored to have perhaps the most advanced EMP program in existence. So if push came to shove, there can be no doubt that the Kremlin has contingency plans of its own to use EMP against the United States. If Russia believed that a nuclear showdown with the United States was imminent for example, the prevailing theory is that Russian leadership would attempt to bypass the consequence of "mutually assured destruction" by launching such a devastating EMP that the U.S. would be knocked out before it could launch a single nuclear missile.

For such a thing to occur, the Russians would indeed have to have a powerful *and very precise* EMP weapon, and they would have to have a great deal of luck to create such a perfect electro magnetic storm that the U.S. is blacked out from coast to coast (they would also have to hope that U.S. nuclear subs wouldn't be able to reach them before being disabled by the pulse). Such unlucky odds for America may seem far fetched, but even the slightest chance of such a negative result needs to be taken into account.

**Chinese Retaliatory Strike**

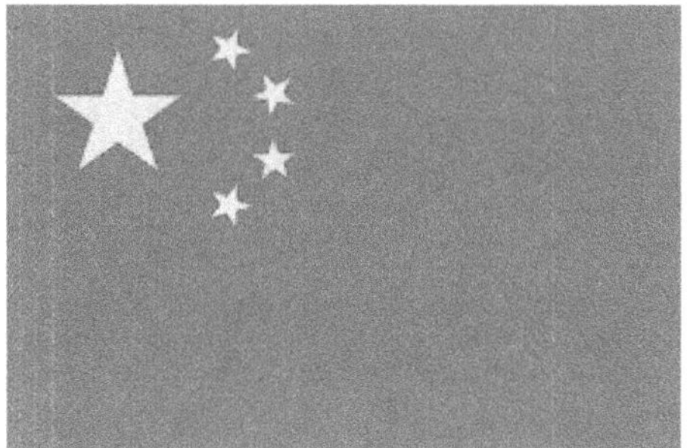

Even in the best of times the United States and China have a rather tenuous relationship. There are quite a few ways that the U.S. and China can rub each other the wrong way and spark a devastating military conflict. For one thing—and as you can see is a common theme in this book—China is loosely allied with North Korea, and in light of the recent threats being leveled by North Korea to the United States, a conflict could erupt that pulls China right along with it.

Just how would such a nightmare scenario occur? Quite easily with the current stance that leader Kim Jong Un of Korea has been taking. Mr. Kim has been persistently pushing the limits of what the United States and the rest of the world can take. The world community is quickly discovering that if they tell Mr. Kim not to do something, in petulant defiance he will do it anyway. He was told not to launch missiles into the Sea of Japan, so he launches two missiles in rapid succession the next day.

And then after making threatening insinuations about attacking the U.S. military outpost of Guam in the middle of the Pacific Ocean, Mr. Kim was sternly warned to "not even think about it". So what does Mr. Kim do? The next day he informs the world media that he won't directly hit Guam—oh no, that would be crazy—but he would like to just set off a huge nuclear bomb right off the coastline instead!

The boyish leader of North Korea is literally testing the waters, pushing and pushing, inch by inch, to see just how far he can take things.

If North Korea did drop a nuclear bomb off the shore of Guam, while it may not lead to direct casualties, obviously the United States could not (without completely losing face and all credibility) stand by and let North Korea get away with blowing up nuclear bombs just outside their harbor! If the U.S. allowed this they would have to allow anything. Then again—if the U.S. does respond to this severe provocation, the crafty North Korean leader could rightfully proclaim that their nuclear test off the shores of Guam didn't technically hurt anyone.

Most would see the flaws in this logic and call this nonsense out for what it was, but push come to shove, China may decide to back its traditional ally. In this scenario, North Korea pushes its luck, takes things way to far, bombs the coast of Guam and forces the U.S. to strike North Korea. China alarmed that its neighbor is being incinerated, and fearing what might happen next, takes the initiative and drops a massive EMP over the U.S. in order to freeze the U.S. assault in its tracks. Let's hope none of this nightmare scenario ever occurs.

North Korea Makes Good on its Threats

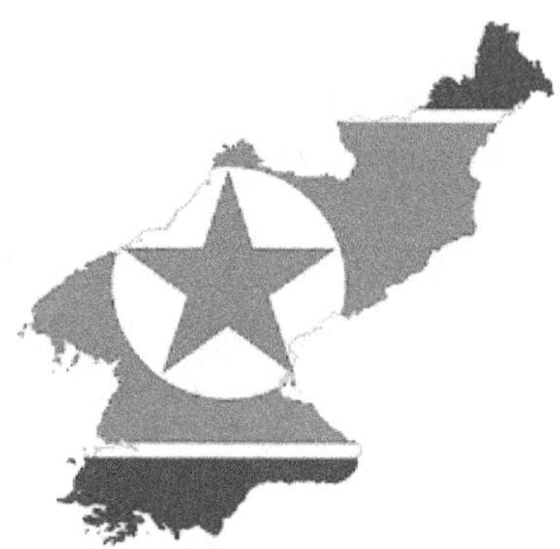

No one quite knows what Kim Jong Un (or as some have dubbed him; the "rocket man") is up to when it comes to his ambitious nuclear missile program. Many have made the claim that the North Korean leader only wishes to have a nuclear deterrent as a safeguard and collateral against any future U.S. attempt at regime change. This argument contends that while non-nuclear countries such as Iraq and Libya have faced grueling regime change either directly or tacitly backed by the United States, nations with nuclear weapons remain safe from such intrusions.

Directly feeding into this belief more than anything else is the glaring fact that the long time dictator of Libya, Momar Kaddafi actually voluntarily turned over his weapons of mass destruction, including the components of a nascent nuclear program with the promise from the Bush administration to never interfere with the Libyan government. But it only took a change of administration a few years later to have President Obama leading the charge to run Kaddafi out of power during the Arab Spring.

If Kaddafi had a nuclear bomb to play as his trump card, this probably never would have happened. It seems that Kim Jong Un has paid attention to this example of a head of state cooperating with nuclear disarmament only to perish, and taken the lesson to heart. This is why for many, it seems that Kim is primarily bluff and bluster, using his nuclear weapons to deter the United States, but would never be crazy enough to actually use them.

But then again, there are many who would point out that if all Kim sought was a nuclear deterrent, all he really needed was one nuclear bomb, just one nuclear weapon is usually enough to deter an outright land invasion of a country, yet Kim kept going after that *one bomb*, he kept going after *two bombs*, and he kept going at *20 bombs*. North Korea is now producing nuclear weapons—and ever more powerful and stronger grade nuclear weapons—at such an exponential rate, that some policy analysts are beginning to sound the alarm that a simple nuclear deterrent is not the only thing Kim is seeking.

For them it seems that Kim is attempting something else entirely. Kim Jong Un seems to have three goals in mind with his nuclear build up; either bully or destroy South Korea and unify the entire Korean peninsula under his reign, get revenge on Japan for the atrocities Japan committed against them during World War Two, and perhaps, just perhaps drop a massive EMP on the United States to make it unable to respond (at least in a timely manner) to North Koreas attacks on its neighbors.

According to this dreadful theory, North Korea would take out the U.S. electrical grid first with a powerful EMP, then bomb, and or flood troops into South Korea, while simultaneously decimating Japan with nuclear and or conventional weapons, hoping that the U.S. would be literally "powerless" to stop them. It is for a scary scenario like this that the U.S. needs to make sure that it can either prevent, or mostly withstand an EMP attack intact, so that North Korea would not be able to make good on its threats.

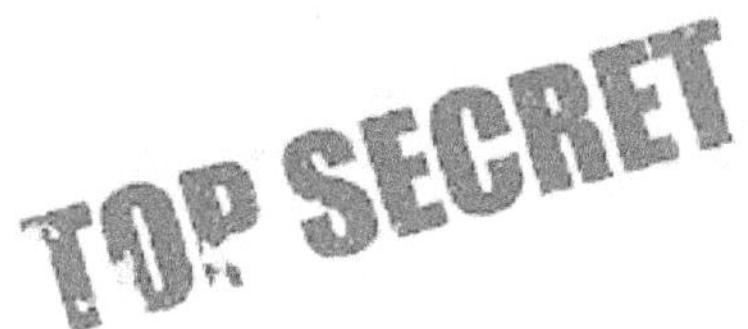

President Barack Obama made a deal with Iran to delay their nuclear program for 10 years, but many skeptical observers believe that Iran is probably continuing their development regardless. Coincidentally enough Iran already has long rage missiles courtesy of North Korea. The fact that North Korea has exported military hardware to Iran is what led President George Bush to make North Korea and Iran, part of what he termed the, "Axis of Evil".

On the surface, the two nations of North Korea and Iran do not have much in common. North Korea is a communist nation that eschews religion while Iran is a hardcore religious state. But despite their diametrically opposed belief systems, both nations have an equal sense of antagonism when it comes to the United States. And this is precisely why the American CIA under the Bush administration had such fear of these two nations actively collaborating with each other.

If Iran secretly produced a bomb, or if North Korea actually colluded with Iran enough to ship them an already constructed weapon, Iran could produce an unpleasant surprise in the form of an EMP burst over the middle of the United States. It would be with terrible irony that the so-called axis of evil would finally live up to all the hype and the fear mongering, by creating an electro magnetic variant of former President Bush's smoking gun.

Terrorists Deploy Suitcase EMP

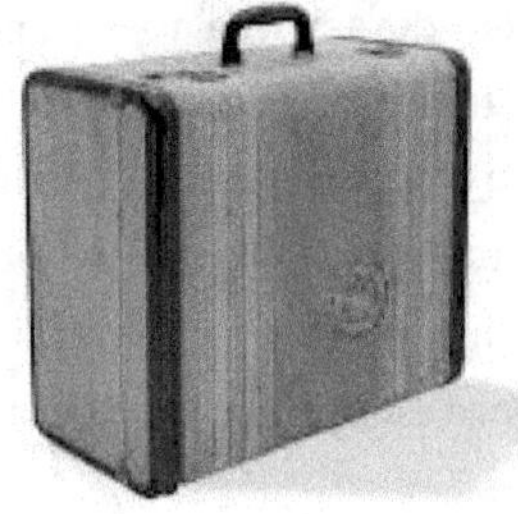

So far in this chapter we have discussed the dangers of other nations subjecting the United States to a nationwide power failure through an EMP attack. Now lets explore the unpleasant possibility of terrorists using a much smaller, so-called "Suitcase EMP" to specifically knock out the power grid of a targeted city. In this scenario a small band of terrorists could unload a suitcase EMP in the middle of downtown New York creating a city-wide blackout.

Not only that, since the infrastructure was so thoroughly fried the terrorists are fully aware that it will take months for city officials to get the power back on. In such an attack, the black out itself would no doubt simply be the first step of the plan, and after the power grid is shut down, the terrorists would then move on to stage to which would be subjecting the disabled city to horrific terrorist attacks through conventional bombings, mass shootings, and even stabbings.

It's an awful thing to think about, but even a small suitcase EMP could lead to such horrible consequences. In order to exact such damage, it is believed that the total cost to finance such a mission—including the gathering of all technical components of the device—would cost less than a couple thousand dollars. A truly sobering statistic, and yet another reason analysts are staying up at night in the never ending struggle to keep the rest of us safe.

Chapter 4: What Defense is there from EMP?

The effects of an EMP are projected to be absolutely devastating to national infrastructure. So the question naturally arises; is there any way to protect against or prevent an EMP strike? As the protectors of a nation, institutions like the United States Pentagon have spent countless hours exploring every possible contingency plan to keep their country out of harms way. And when it comes to an EMP attack, many different contingencies for defense and preservation of the nation have been explored.

But it isn't just those on the national level that should carry the entire burden, each and every one of us as citizens should also be educated as much as possible on the means of our own survival. Having that said, this chapter uses a dual approach describing how the government as well as the individual citizen may be able to defend against the onslaught of an EMP.

Metallic Shielding

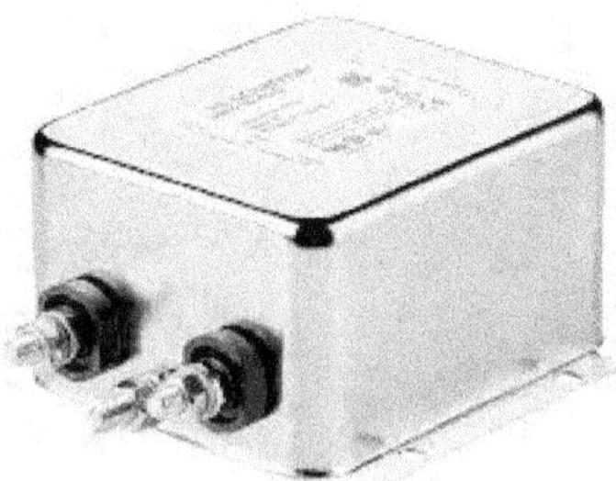

In order to use metallic shielding on electrical equipment, you will need to use a continuous piece of shielding such as copper or steel would provide. These metal shields usually don't completely cover the interior however, and will most likely consist of some exceedingly small holes for ventilation. Additional, auxiliary materials are usually used in order to compensate for this perceived gap in security. The shielding should be about half a millimeter thick in order to provide the best protection from the blast of an electromagnetic pulse.

<u>Tailored Hardening</u>

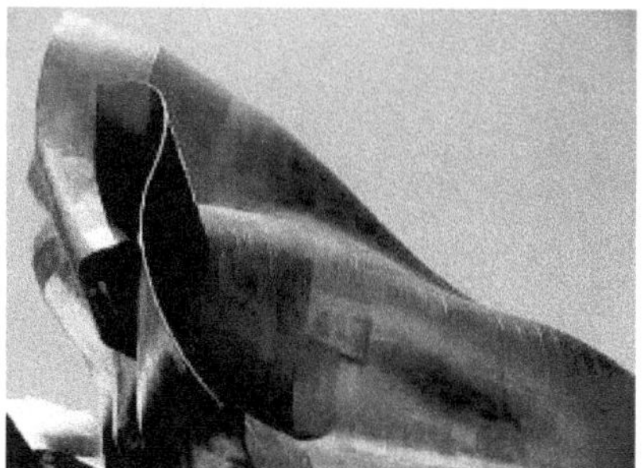

When it comes to tailor made hardening of electrical equipment in defense of a potential EMP attack, the first thing that needs to be considered is whether or not the system itself will be viable if hardening is achieved. With tailor hardening you are only encasing the most sensitive pieces of the electronics in metal cases. Being able to differentiate what part of an appliance or device needs hardening and what parts could do without is crucial in keeping an EMP defense within budget. But although this method is cheaper it has not proven to be quite as reliable as complete metallic shielding.

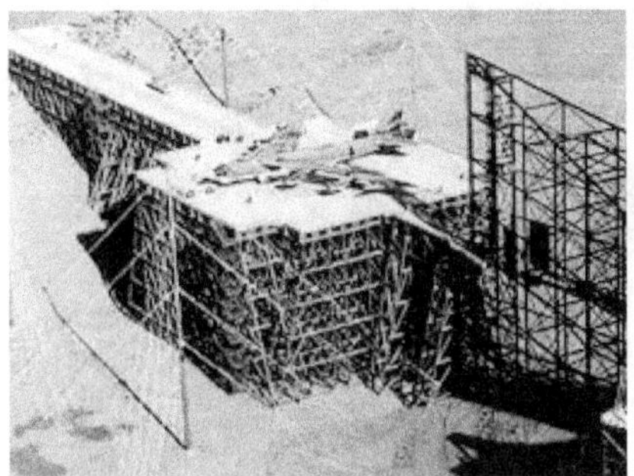

Many have attempted to claim that there is not contingency plan when it comes to private sector infrastructure. This couldn't be further from the truth. Since civil infrastructure of the private sector could be severely damaged, measures have been taken to put into place powerful surge protectors that could not only withstand a bolt of lighting, but could also take on an electromagnetic pulse. This is a step in the right direction, but these surge protectors are by no means full proof and could easily be overwhelmed, but it is at least a start when it comes to preparing the private sector.

Detecting and Knocking out An EMP Device

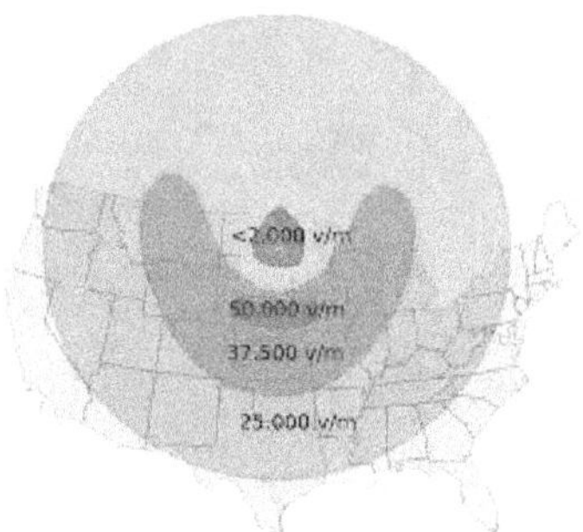

In recent years, primarily due to provocations from North Korea, the U.S. has stepped up its efforts to perfect methods of shooting down nuclear missiles and other offensive weapons, in mid flight. The conventional method is to use offensive missiles such as the "patriot" class interceptors to aim, shoot, and knock enemy missiles out of the sky. In addition to this, there are also projects in the works with laser technology to shoot down incoming objects.

The U.S. military has prototypes of ground laser batteries as well as continued research into space based laser platforms as was touted in Ronald Reagan's "Strategic Defense Initiative" program of the 1980's. And when it comes to something more subtle such as a suitcase EMP that terrorists are attempting to deploy in the middle of a city, man's best friend may be his dog after all.

There are several programs that have successfully trained the miraculous nose of the common dog to find and ferret out the components of what would make up an EMP device. So whether its through a patriot missile, a ground based laser, Ronald Reagan's SDI, or your dog's trusty sniffer, there are ways to detect and potentially knock out an EMP device.

Chapter 5: Important Food and Medical Supplies

Although there is not much the individual citizen can do if their power grid is knocked down—to turn the power back on—there are several other life saving aspects you can thoroughly prepare for. First and foremost on your list of preparation for an EMP attack would be adequate food and medical supplies.

Due to the nature of the crisis, these supplies would have to be completely nonperishable items that you could leave out in the item or packed away in boxes without any damage to the contents of the supplies. In this chapter we will explore some of the best of these nonperishable food and medical supplies to have on hand in the event of an EMP blast.

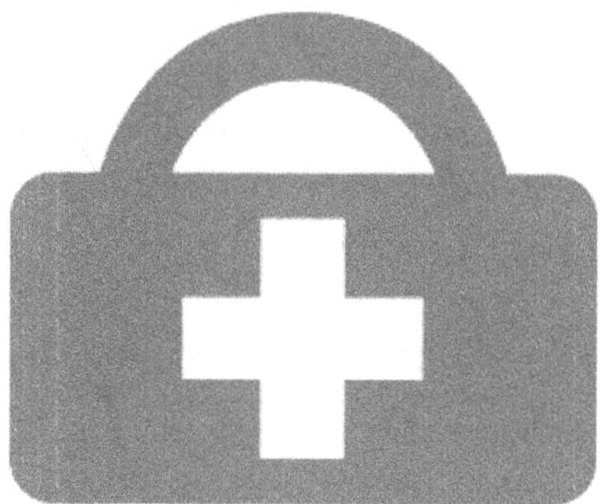

This is prepping 101 for just about any disaster, but yes, in the event of an EMP the traditional First Aid Kit would be a tremendous resource to have available. You should have a fully stocked kit with such medical supply staples such as cold packs, hydrogen peroxide, some Tylenol, and most importantly, needle, thread, and scissors. The latter items are of extreme import if you have to sow your own stitches. It may not always be pretty, but basic supplies like these will help you to survive the aftermath of an EMP blast.

Garlic

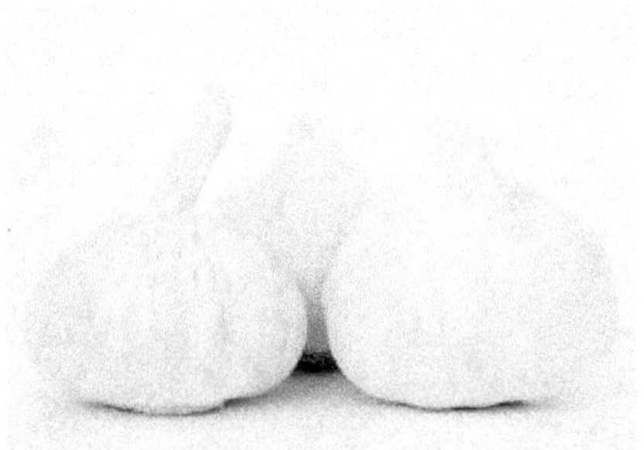

This herb is good to eat and heal your wounds at the same time! You probably recognize Garlic more for its use as a seasoning, but if you were to sprinkle a little bit of it in your wounds, it would work to greatly ease your pain and speed up the healing process. Garlic has special compounds that help to promote blood clotting and promote the formation of new platelets at the sight of the injury helping it to scab over and heal much faster than it would otherwise. So be sure to pack some garlic!

Gauze

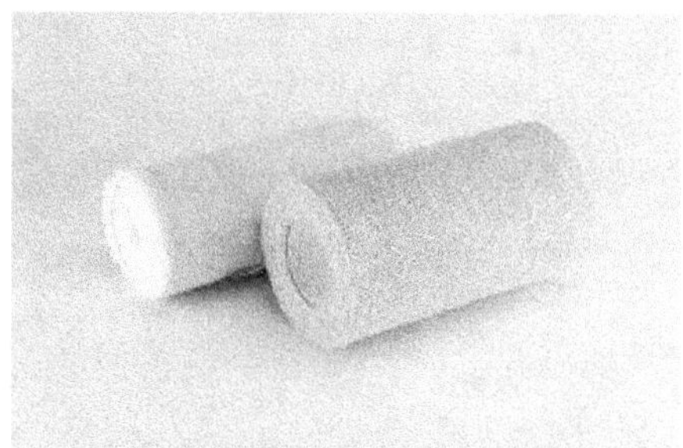

The aftermath of an EMP can be a hazardous place, especially at night when it is difficult to see. These extra risk factors could lead to all kinds of injuries. This is why having a good roll of gauze on hand is critical to offset the danger. Immediately after you get injured wrap up the injury up with gauze and allow the area to pressurize in place so that it can heal. Gauze is an important medical supply to have.

Canned Goods

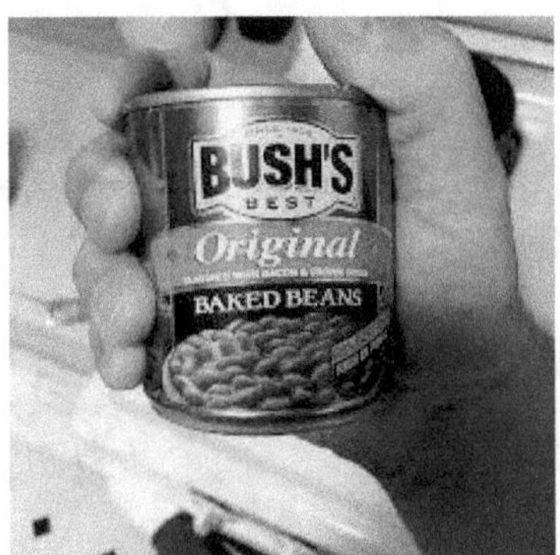

Some of the best food you could ever have stashed away in your cupboards are canned goods. These cans of food can last for decades. So yes, even though you may have laughed at your crazy uncle who kept a large supply of emergency canned goods big enough to fill a walk in closet, in our uncertain world such a practice is completely reasonable. In the face of an EMP attack when food might become incredibly scarce, such things don't seem quite so ridiculous! So yes, stock up on your canned goods!

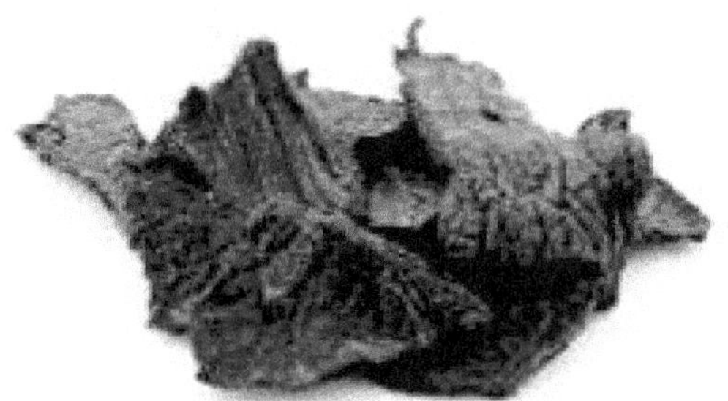

Beef Jerky and other dried out meat are not just a good snack; they are a marvelous lifeline of protein preservation! Beyond beef jerky, just about any meat can be dried out with the right combination of salty brine, and through established drying techniques. If you don't know how to do it yourself, you can always purchase a nice supply of already dried beef and otherwise jerky! It's a great foodstuff to help see you through the worst of an EMP!

Conclusion: Surviving an Electro Magnetic Pulse

It is definitely a scary thing to wake up and find your entire city block out of power. It is horrifying then to find that you can't even start your car to flee the scene! But these are the startling realities of an EMP attack. In the chance that some rogue actor decides to implement such a devious strike against us, we have to be vigilant and we have to be prepared. I hope this book has left you just a little bit more informed, and more importantly reassured, of how you can survive an electromagnetic pulse. Thank you for reading!

SURVIVAL MEDICINE

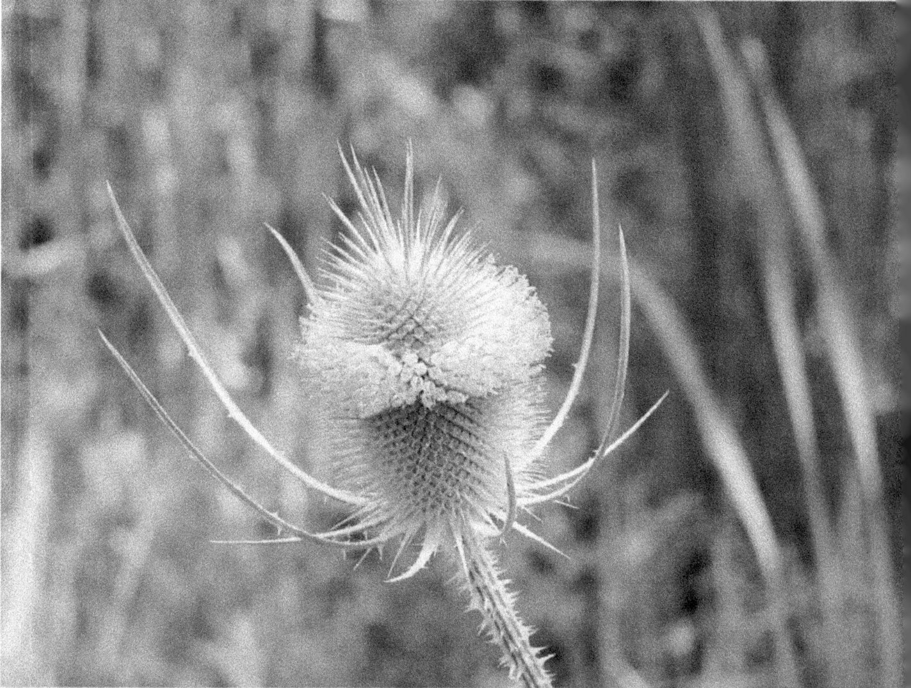

30 Best Essential Oils, Healing Herbs
And Salves For Excellent Health
+ 22 Effective Natural
Remedies For The Treatment Of Diseases

CRYSTAL WILKINS

Survival Medicine:

30 Best Essential Oils, Healing Herbs And Salves For Excellent Health + 22 Effective Natural Remedies For The Treatment Of Diseases

Introduction

Health is intrinsically linked with everything we do. If you can keep yourself in the right physical state, you will be much better predisposed to be in the right mental state. So it is that the basics of our health are the basis of happiness itself. If you want to be healthy both mind and body in order to survive an emergency, let's get down to the basics of health!

Preparing for the unpredictable is not an oxymoron it is simply being proactive in a troubled world. And in any crisis situation our health should be of number one concern to us.

One of the most important things before picking the right survival medicine is to have the basic knowledge about its usage. It is really important that you identify herbs correctly. We have provided photographs of most of these herbs and have added additional information about their appearance so that you can hand-pick the natural herbs of your choice.

After when you have identified the natural products that can help you survive, the second most important factor is regarding their correct usage. We have listed the most appropriate way to use these herbs and how they can help you in various ways. A proper listing of their benefits has been provided so that you can figure out how and when to use these herbs correctly.

A single herb can be of numerous usages and you should certainly keep a few of them with you when you move, as an unforeseen disaster might come unannounced. A wide range of natural herbs have been discussed in the guide – from edible products to antiseptic ones, anti-inflammatory herbs to plants that can help in skin treatment, and more.

Health is intrinsically linked with everything we do. If you can keep yourself in the right physical state, you will be much better predisposed to be in the right mental state. So it is that the basics of our health are the basis of happiness itself. If you want to be healthy both mind and body in order to survive an emergency, let's get down to the basics of Survival Medicine!

First Aid is not only for lifesaving purposes, it is also an invaluable tool for managing everyday injuries and illnesses that can occur in your home or any other environment. Interestingly, the numbers of injuries that take place in the home are staggering when compared to those that occur in other places.

Think of the times you may have tripped and fallen over the cat, burnt yourself cooking, struck your thumb with a hammer during home maintenance, or simply spent too much time out in the sun mowing your lawn. And if you have children, the numbers of at home injuries increase dramatically!

Knowing the basics of first aid is also essential if you plan on doing any outdoor excursions, particularly in the wilderness or out on the water. There, you can face a lot of hidden dangers that don't exist in your urban neighborhood, and it is much harder to dash to the emergency room or get paramedic help. In those types of situations, survival is down to you.

Being prepared for any scenario can increase your chances of survival. This is also true of natural disasters, as these can strike at any time without any warning. Tornados, hurricanes, earthquakes, are all extreme forces of nature, and loss of life is a very real possibility, so if you know first aid, not only can you help yourself and your family, but also you're neighbors, and the greater community. Your skills would be invaluable in these types of situations. But first, you need to know how to assess a situation.

Steps to Properly Assess the Situation

Step 1: Minimize Risk

The number one priority in any emergency situation is to first ensure that you as the rescuer are not in any danger. Look around the area and check that whatever caused the injury is no longer a threat. Do not put yourself at risk, or you too could become a victim, which then leaves nobody to assist.

Step 2: Primary Assessment

This is where you check the airway, breathing and circulation of the victim. Note whether or not the victim is breathing, and how they are breathing. You may need to explore the mouth with your fingers to see if there is an obstruction of the airway.

Next, check the circulation by feeling for a pulse either on the neck, the inside of the wrist, or if necessary the groin.

The next part of the assessment is to check whether or not there is an injury to the spinal cord. If this type of injury is suspected, the person should not be moved, and the neck must be supported at all times.

Also note the temperature of the environment, particularly if it is very hot or very cold, as this could have a huge impact on the victim. If they can't be moved, cover them with something to keep them warm, or create a shield from the heat using whatever is nearby and available.

Step 3: Secondary Assessment

Once you have ascertained the victim is breathing and has a pulse, the next step in the assessment process is to determine whether or not there are injuries. This could involve speaking to the victim if they are conscious and asking where they are feeling any pain. If the victim is unconscious, you will need to check for injuries by gently feeling and looking at the body from the head to the toes.

At this point you will also be checking for any discoloration, such as blueness or pale color of the face which may indicate an internal issue such as shock.

First Aid Basics

DRSABCD

DRSABCD is a formula that is taught to anyone learning first aid. This acronym is important to remember, as it will help you follow the correct procedures when faced with an emergency medical situation. The acronym stands for:

D – Danger

Check that there is no further risk or danger to yourself first, then the others around you including the injured or sick person.

R – Response

Note whether or not the person is conscious or responds to your voice or touch.

S – Send for Help

If possible, call emergency services, or if necessary, send someone to get help.

A – Airway

Check the airway and make sure it is clear of any obstruction.

B – Breathing

Look to see if the chest is moving up and down as it would during breathing. Alternatively, listen to their breath sounds near the mouth or nose.

C – Cardiopulmonary Resuscitation (CPR)

If the victim is not breathing and is unconscious, begin CPR.

D – Defibrillate

If a defibrillation device is available, and the situation requires it, use it.

Chapter 1. Aromatherapy as Survival Medicine

Aromatherapy is an ancient practice with powerful results for modern survival medicine. Just take a look at the following examples and how they can greatly enrich your life—no matter the situation.

Frankincense Oil

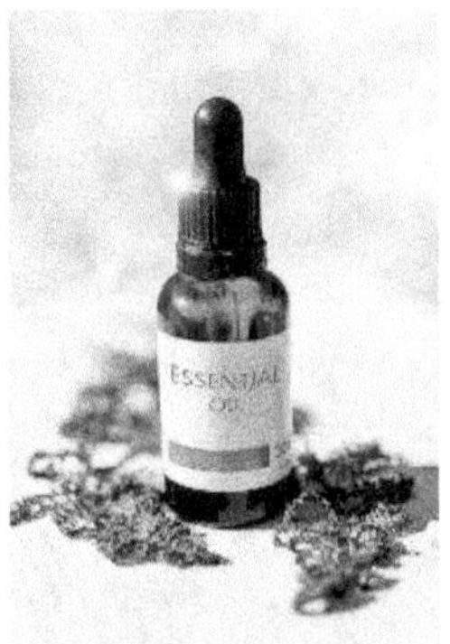

Frankincense has a long history of use. It was prized in ancient times both for its alluring aroma and for its healing properties. Just rub this essential oil into the skin and the healing properties of this herb will work to holistically treat your entire body. It boosts the immune system and cleanses at the same time.

In order to administer Frankincense Oil, either breathe in the aroma from a fresh bottle of essential oil or place a few drops in an incense burner and let the aroma fill the entire room, so that you can benefit from the treatment gradually as you go about your day.

Jasmine Oil

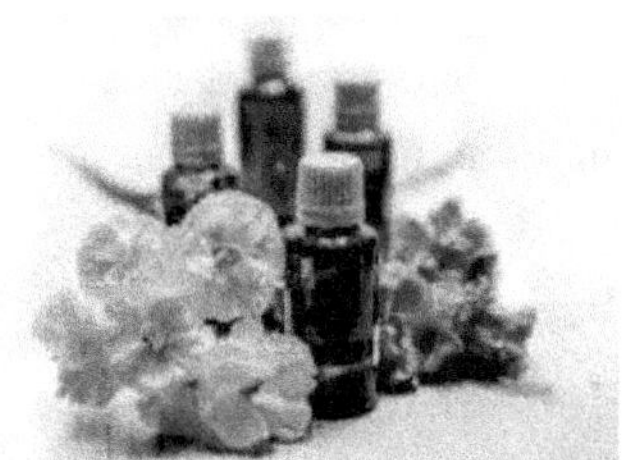

Jasmine has quite a lovely aroma and most that have breathed it in will agree to how refreshing it can be. And when you concentrate the oil of jasmine down to its most powerful form for aroma therapy the effects can be downright life changing. This essential oil has been known to boost memory and overall mental focus for those that use it. Just breathe in a few drops of this stuff and you will know the true meaning of aromatherapy for survival medicine.

Peppermint Oil

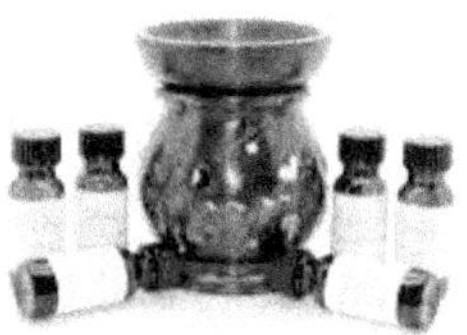

This refreshing blast of peppermint will help to calm your nerves and maybe even boost your metabolism! Peppermint is also known to open up the breathing passages so if you are having any trouble with congestion of shortness of breath, you may want to seriously give peppermint a try. As an asthma sufferer myself I can attest to the healing power of peppermint. Just a few whiffs of this stuff and I am all better. So be sure to keep some of this wondrous healing herb on hand for your own survival medicine.

Coriander Oil

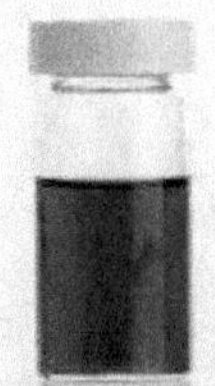

I was first exposed to coriander oil as something to cook with. But little did I know that coriander oil is also great for aromatherapy. Just by breathing in the aroma of this oil you will be able to greatly increase the blood supply of your cardiovascular system. This extra burst of blood flow will actually help your body to relax considerably. So if you feel like may need a break, just breathe in some coriander oil.

Grapefruit Oil

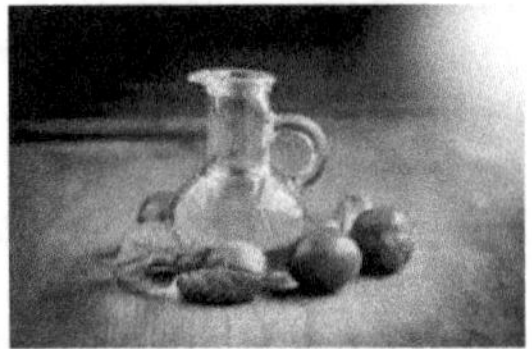

The powerful aromatherapy provided by grapefruit oil can work to really get you going in the morning! This essential oil when breathed in directly will allow for your body to get that extra boost it needs to get through the day. Regular regimens of breathing in this oil could also greatly improve your mental clarity and recall of events. So yes, I would advise, if you need survival medicine, then you need to give some grapefruit oil a try!

Neola Oil

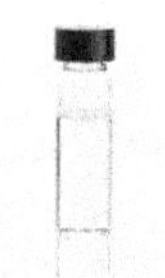

The effect of this essential oil when breathed into the body through a regular routine of aromatherapy is almost immediate. As soon as you breathe it in you will begin to feel your heart beat just a little bit slower. And after your treatment progresses your whole body will soon be relaxed! Neola oil is highly recommended!

Cyprus Oil

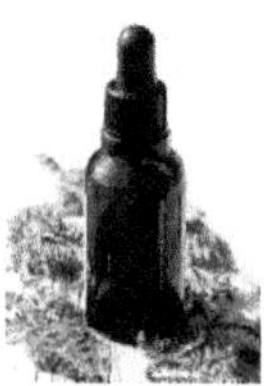

You may have noticed the scent of cypress in many cars you have been driven in since Cyprus is the number one scent in car air fresheners. You may have had the privilege of sitting under a tree shaped car air freshener and breathed in that tree-like scent. Well this essential oil is also quite effective as a form of aromatic treatment for a wide range of illnesses and discomforts.

Most notably this aromatic oil is great for giving those who breathe it in a refreshing calm and an increase in overall energy. So if you need a bit of a boost at any time during yo9ur day you should just take some time to stop and smell the Cyprus!

Chapter 2. Herbs as Survival Medicine

Milk Thistle

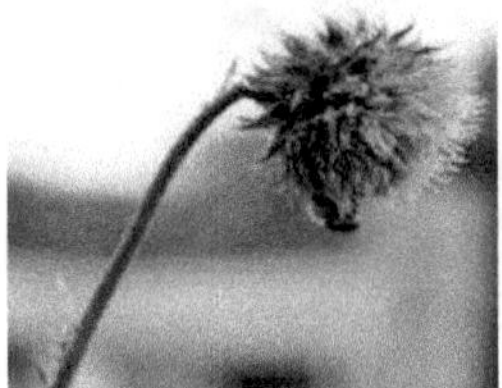

This herb is another great item to pack in your medicine chest. With its ability to reduce inflammation, this herb has been known to have some rather amazing results. Milk thistle serves to boost liver function and in some instances has even been seen to reverse the effects of cirrhosis. If you have any inflammation whatsoever, simply apply some Milk Thistle directly to the area afflicted and you will see results.

Red Clover

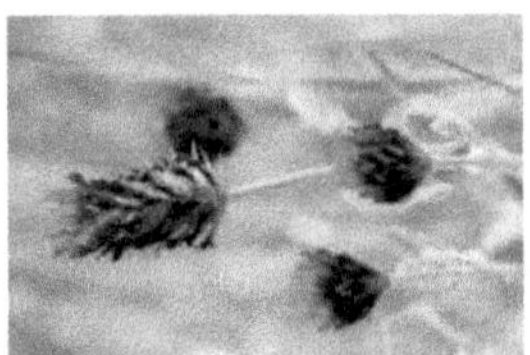

Red Clover is a powerful herbal antibiotic that can greatly boost the immune system. This herb has even been known to increase the red blood cell count in those that use it. Interestingly enough, Red Clover is also a natural anticoagulant and can loosen up blood clots in rather rapid fashion. This in turn provides a general boost in health no matter what you may be facing.

Yarrow

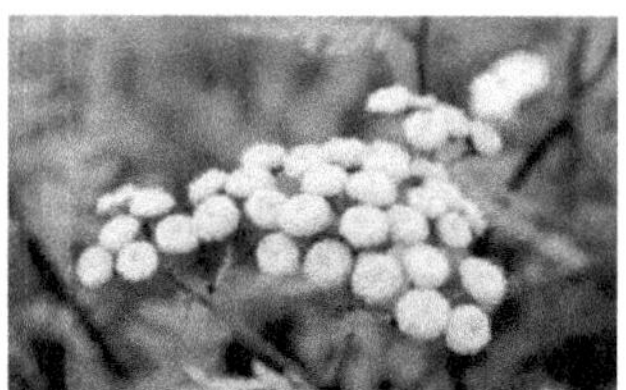

Yarrow is an herb that has been used for centuries; and with good reason. This herb can get to work on inflammation and congestion in the human body, almost immediately. This herbal antibiotic also works well against injuries, and as soon as it is applied to an injured site, it gets to work cleansing the injury and promoting the formation for blood platelets for a quick and effective healing.

Gauche

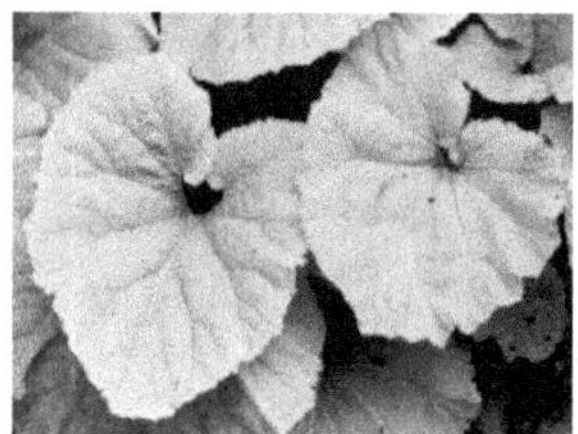

This herb is a great antibiotic fighter and its best work is done to reduce inflammation and boost the immune system. Just apply a small amount of this herbal antibiotic to the skin and you will be able to enhance your body's ability to stand up to and survive all manner of airborne illnesses. Give this herbal Gauche Antibiotic a try!

Ginkgo

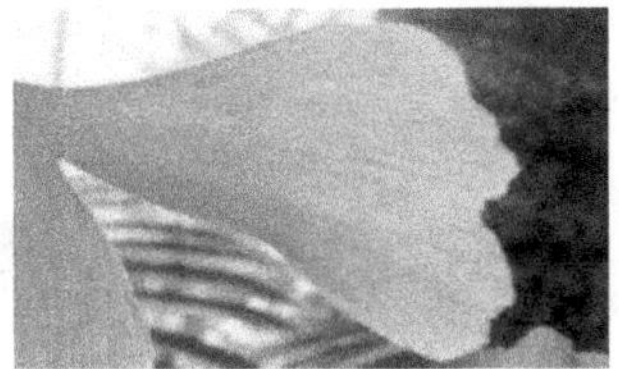

Ginkgo is a powerful and useful allergy fighter and works to reduce inflammation. This herb is also great when it comes to improving the flow of oxygen to the brain. It is for this reason that so many take Ginkgo to boost their memory and concentration. So if you are feeling at all slow and sluggish in the morning—or any other time for that matter—a good dose of Ginkgo tea could really do you some good! This tea can be made through either boiling powdered Ginkgo or raw Ginkgo leaves.

Anise

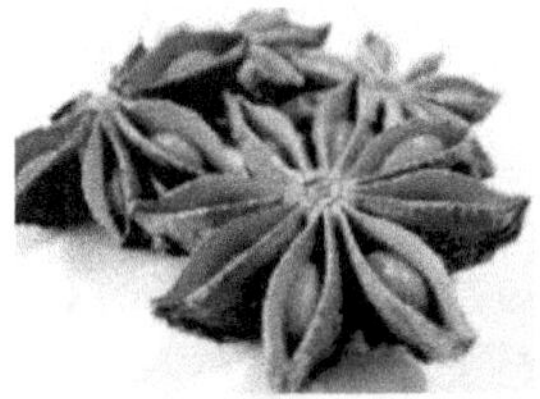

This herb works out just great as an herbal antibiotic, killing most bacteria right on the spot. This herbal antibiotic also works on the urinary system, helping to clear up any incontinence that someone may be facing, and putting the whole body into a kind of detox, almost immediately. One of the best ways to administer this healing herb is to boil it into a nice and tasty tea. So drink up folks because this Herbal Anise is on me!

Chervil

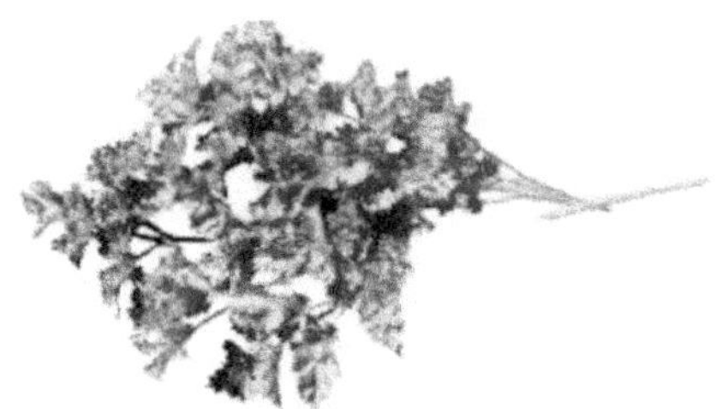

Chervil has a real proven ability when it comes to killing bacteria, getting rid of headaches and calming upset stomachs. It is the latter from which many a camper has benefited. It is common practice for many survivalists to simply pop a leaf of chervil in their mouth and chew in order to relieve their upset stomach. I have tried this myself and can say that it really does wonders.

Cloves

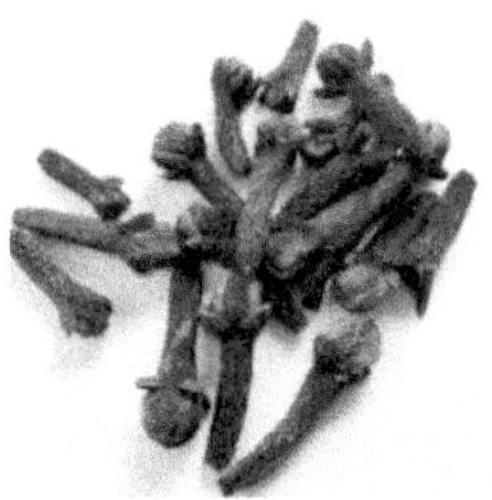

In a similar fashion to chervil, cloves have been placed directly into the mouth of many dental patients in order to kill bacteria and curb inflammatory agents. This herb also works as a mild form of pain reliever and can be used to successfully numb up a bad toothache if needed.

Sage

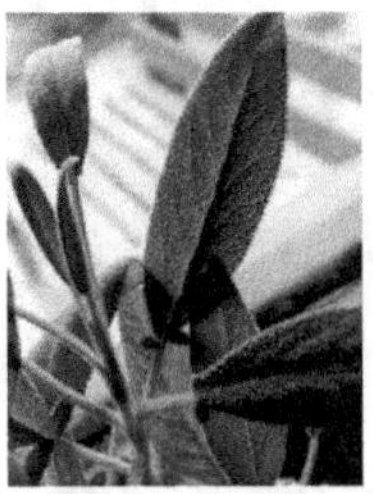

This medicinal herb takes survival medicine to a whole new live in the way that it can successfully reduce all manner of pain and kill bacterial infections on the spot. If you have fallen and sustained an injury, just a very small application of this healing herb will work to alleviate any pain that you may feel. Another great benefit of herbal sage is its ability to treat asthma. I have suffered with asthma most of my life myself, and applications of this herb have helped to improve my own breathing considerably when I have tried it.

Valerian

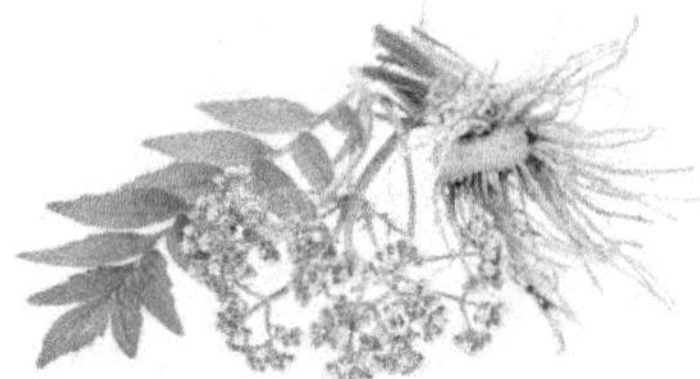

Valerian is also another very popular nighttime home remedies to deal with your anxiety. It contains some elements of mild tranquilizing properties that will almost guarantee you and will get you a good night sleep. However, without all dreaded and the weird hangover feeling early in the morning that you may sometimes have to get with some other pharmaceuticals.

Passionflower

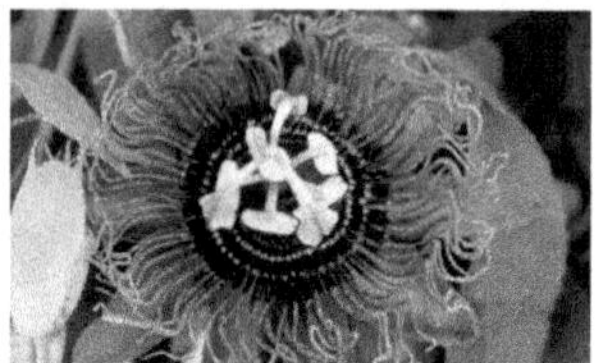

Passionflower is also referred to as folk for a natural remedy and anxiety, insomnia and panic attacks. Passionflower has been shown in many studies to treat anxiety is a very remarkably well.

One study has found it has to be as effective as benzodiazepine drugs, but the only difference is without the drowsiness. Passionflower may also help you to feel an emotionally balanced and exceptionally beneficial way.

Nonetheless, if you suffer from exaggerated emotions then this is by far one of the most efficient home remedies to deal with anxiety, and it needs to be part of your daily regimen.

Lemon Balm

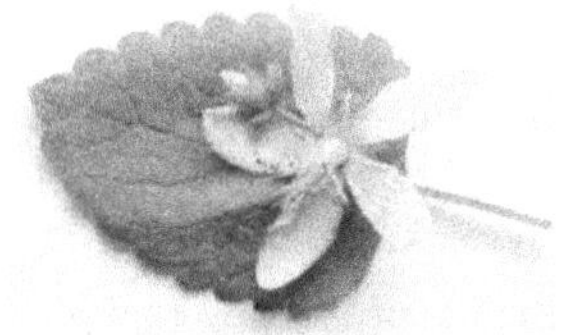

Lemon Balm also is known as 'Melissa officinalis' which is one herbal supplement and tea to treat anxiety and calm your nerves.

Some studies suggested that the use of lemon balm can decrease insomnia, anxiety, hyper excitation and fatigue.

 A lemon balm extract which should be taken 300mg at breakfast and 300mg at dinner too which may help reduced insomnia mainly due to a decrease in nervousness and also to decreased agitation, guilt, hyper excitation and fatigue too.

California poppy

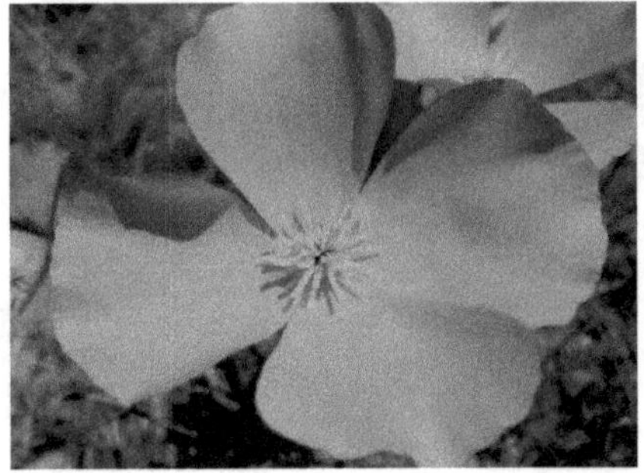

California poppy also called Eschscholtzia californica, which is a tension-relieving, anti-anxiety, sedative, and antispasmodic herb. California poppy also helps with sleeplessness and quells a headache as well as muscular spasm from stress. Some gentle and non-addictive actions are much safer for children and the elderly.

Wild Lettuce

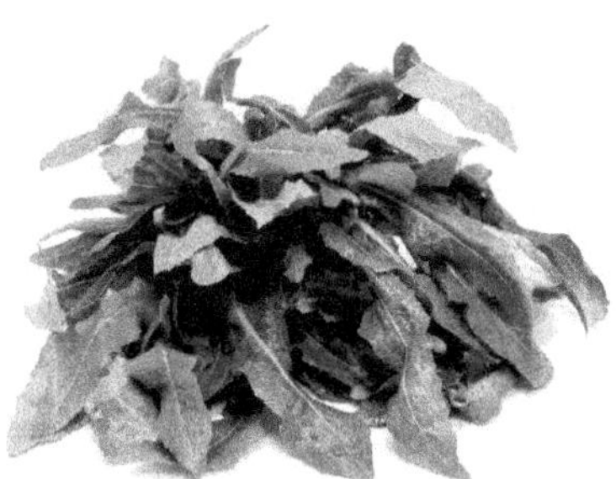

Wild Lettuce is of the species of lactic vireos, which is a mild tranquilizer that may be used for calming a nervous or overactive nervous system. It is very suitable for anxious children or even adolescents. It majorly helps with insomnia. It is also a general pain reliever and antispasmodic that can primarily be used for short coughs.

Rosemary

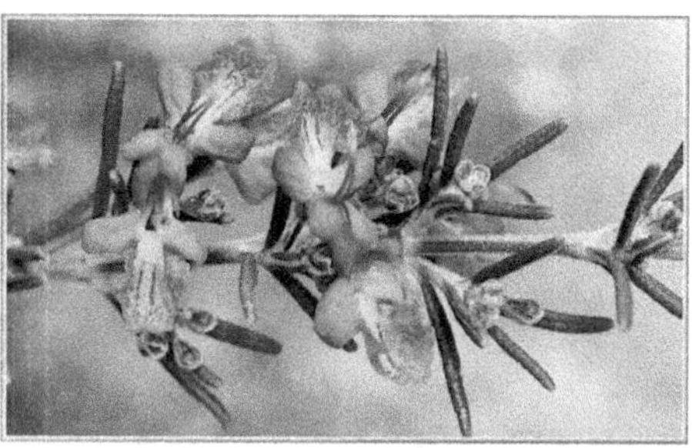

The herb that makes chicken sing and soups taste wonderful helps treat headaches, nervous tension, a nervous stomach, cleanse the face, and can even help to stimulate hair growth. Great in teas, oils, and soaks.

Chapter 3. Soothing Survival Salves

Here are a few healing salves that will help you survive just about anything that comes your way!

Almond Lip Salve

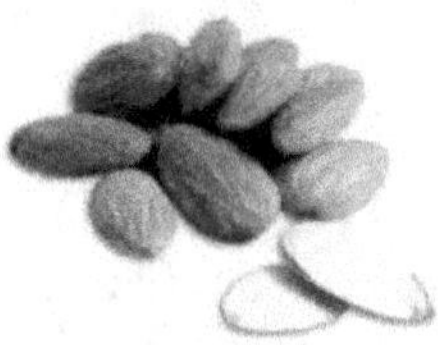

This healing salve is a natural way to cure dry lips. If you have repeatedly dry and cracking lips you can greatly benefit by even the smallest of applications of this herbal lip balm. This lip balm is almost odorless and has just a slightly sweet taste that will not interfere with eating or anything else you do throughout the course of a day.

Coconut Salve

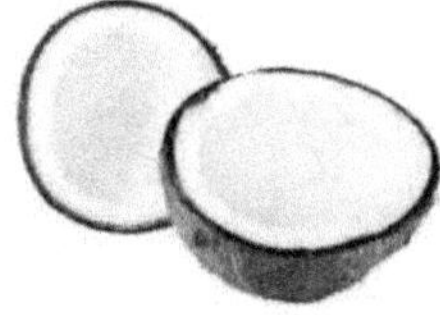

Coconut salves are always classy and soothing. This salve is no exception. Made out of concentrated coconut oil, just a little dab will do you! Place this coconut salve on your lips, feet, arms, or any other part of your being that could use just a little bit of soothing!

Lemon Balm Salve

Lemon Balm is perhaps one of the most popular salves that you could ever use. These salves are great for chapped lips and even better for rough hands. You can also use this salve as an herbal antibiotic since lemon naturally kills all germs and bacteria on contact. Lemon balm salve is also great for the face and even small applications of it can help can clear up complexions and even treat wrinkling of the skin.

Cat's Claw Salve

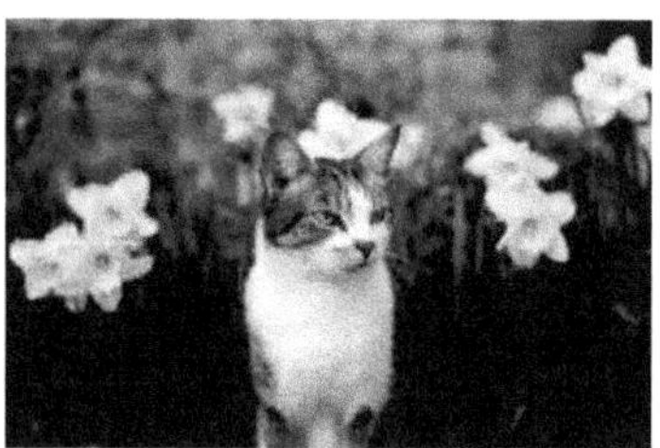

This healing salve is a great immune booster and can even help promote the production of white blood cells when regularly applied to the skin. Simply put; external viruses, bacteria, and other germs don't stand a chance when cat's claw is applied!

Burdock Root

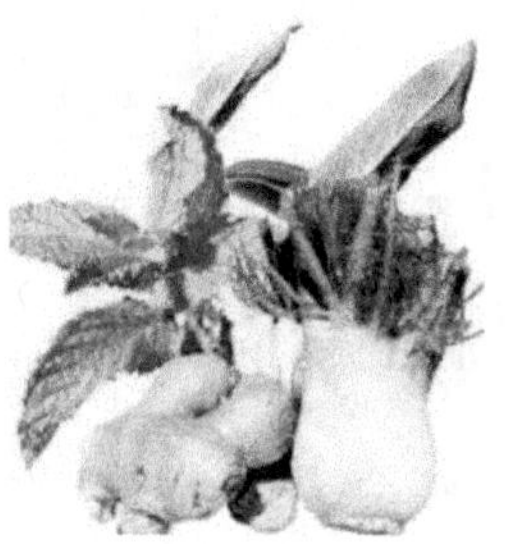

If you are suffering from arthritis, the inflammation fighting power of a little Burdock Root could be just what the doctor ordered for you. Just a brief application of this healing salve and your arthritis will be long behind you. Be sure to pack this herbal healing salve in your bag as part of your survival medicine arsenal.

Aloe Vera

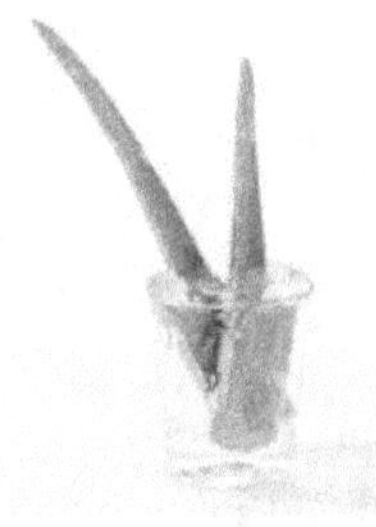

Burns have met their match with Aloe Vera. This healing salve sooths even as it protects. As soon as you apply Aloe Vera to a burn on the skin you will feel the soothing relief that this herb can provide. Burns by their nature—as well as damaging tissue structure—take all of the moisture out of the injury.

But an application of Aloe Vera will put that moisture back in. So don't hesitate to bring yourself some Aloe Vera folks!

The best way to pack it is in a tube, but *if you can hack it*, you can make some of your own. All you have to do is take the Aloe Vera leaf, split it open and then scoop the gel out. Either way you will have a powerful and soothing herbal healing salve on your hands.

<u>Dandelion</u>

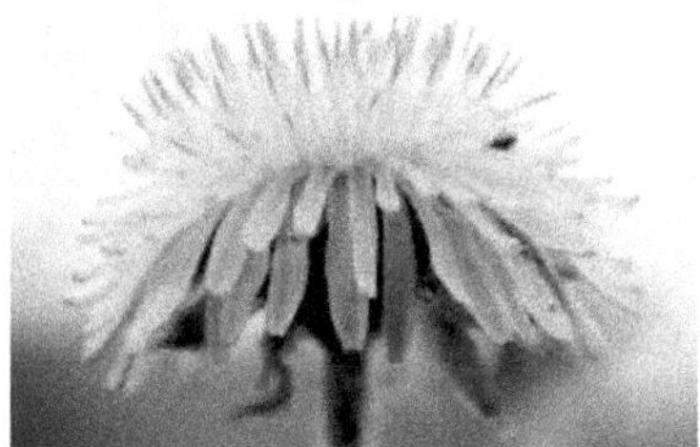

Dandelions are quite prolific, you see than sprouting up in yards, parking lots and businesses all across the country. The bane of lawnmowers and weed whackers everywhere—these little yellow guys really do get around.

And this healing salve once applied can do wonders for everything from allergies to immune system protection. Improving the production of platelets in the blood, this healing salve has been shown to even improve the lives of cancer patients. So this is definitely a survival medicine tat could be of some great use for you.

Ashwagandha

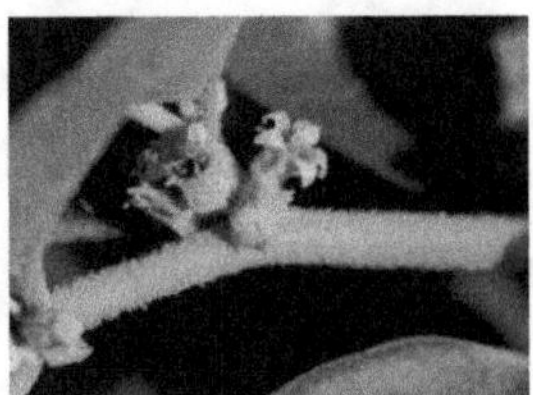

This healing salve has been with us for quite some time, and known as an "adaptogen" it can work to adapt to just about any situation that is thrown at it. Ashwagandha can help with everything from inflammation, to boosting immune health, to healing injuries from cuts, scrapes, and burns. All of this makes for some great soothing survival salves!

Chapter 4. Diseases And Their Remedies

Heartburn

This is an over production of stomach acids to different degrees. Many antacids on the market can make this worse instead of better, leading to a complete dependence to the medication.

Here are some simple things you can do to help when it flares up:

● Parsley helps to curve heartburn. Chewing on a sprig will release the juice and stem the acid flow.

● Peppermint tea will help cool the burn.

Heartburn Tea

1 tsp Peppermint
(cools the core)
1 tsp Chamomile Flowers
1 tsp Lemon Balm leaves cut
(helps curve acid)
Drink cold

Marshmallow and Chamomile syrup

1 Ounce Marshmallow Root
(helps to absorb acids)
1 Ounce Chamomile Flowers
(calms the stomach)
2 Ounces Raw Honey
1 Tbsp every four to six hours.

Upset Stomach

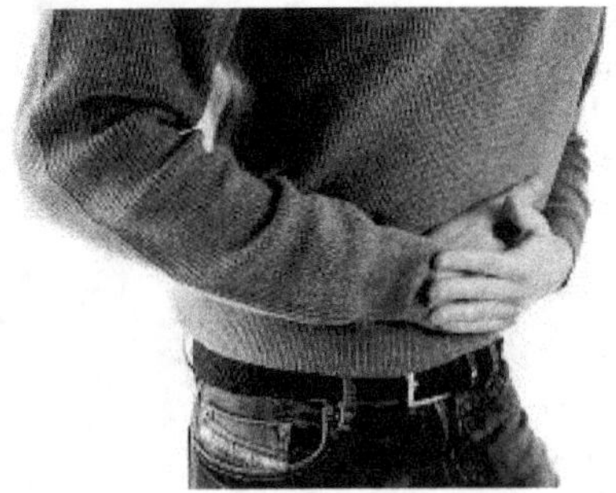

This can be as small as an upset stomach to nausea and vomiting. Here are couple of things you can try:

• Chewing on a clove and swallowing the juice will alleviate nausea

• Putting a small amount of Allspice powder under your tongue will do the same.

Calming Tummy Tea

1 tsp Chamomile Flowers
1 tsp Peppermint leaves
1 tsp Fennel Seeds
(soothes the stomach)

Calming Tummy Syrup

1/2 ounce Peppermint Leaves
1/2 ounce Fennel Seeds
1/2 ounce Anise Seeds
1/2 ounce Lavender flowers
2 ounces raw honey

Nervous System

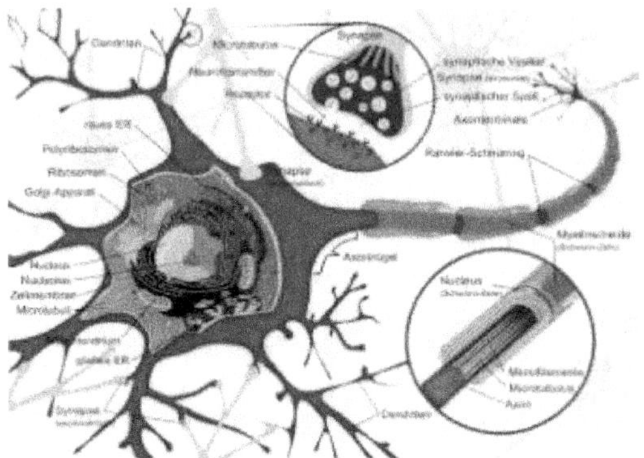

Made of our brain, eyes, spinal cord, and millions of synapses that fire off in order to deliver information to the brain the nervous system is truly a marvel, and many biologist have yet to unlock all its mysteries, but there are some ailments that are prevalent today which herbs to can help stem, if not help cure.

Alzheimer's Disease

Given a name in the late 80's this disease causes dementia in a patient, often reverting them back to child-like behavior and erasing memories of past experiences and even loved ones. There have been many reports of patients wandering off or family members getting in a car and driving only to not realize where they are.

Gingko Biloba has been tested, and in double blind studies has shown it can reverse early stages of Alzheimer's and lessen the severity of later stages.

Senility

This is quite different from dementia. Instead of wandering off or losing memories, it begins to present itself as being absent-minded and not able to recall things right away. This is simply due to the fact we need more B vitamins as we get older to help our brain function at the levels we are used to and for our nervous systems to function as they should.

Tea for concentration

1 tsp Peppermint leaves
1 tsp Gingko Bilboa
1 tsp Kelp (for B vitamins)

Extract for concentration

1 ounce Peppermint
1 ounce Kelp
1 ounce Gingko Biloba
1 ounce Gotu Kola
(Does the same thing as Gingko)

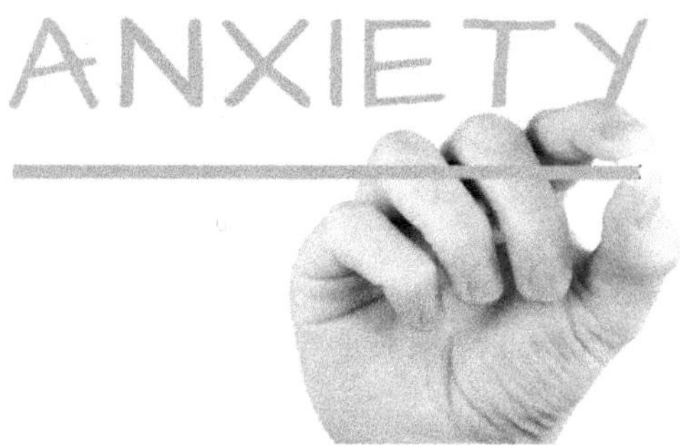

Anxiety can be debilitating. It can completely cripple someone leaving them unable to function. Here are couple of remedies that can help.

Nerve Tea

1 tsp Chamomile Flowers
1 tsp Catnip leaves
1 tsp Lavender Flowers

Herbal Bath

1/2 Ounce Lavender Flowers
1/2 Ounce Chamomile Flowers

Depression

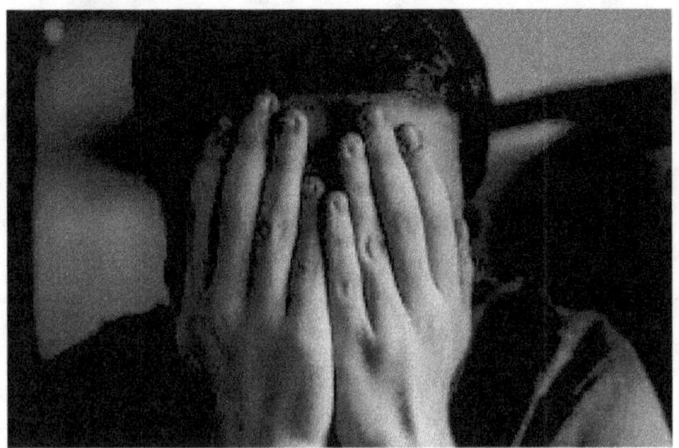

Many people suffer from depression. It can take hours out of the day from your life by making you feel lethargic, and uninterested in everyday things. Just keep in mind, if you are bi-polar, you will have seek further advice from a licensed physician. The same goes for depression caused by chemical imbalances.

Saint John's Wort is the best herb to take for depression provided you are not already taking anti-depression medication.

<u>***Arthritis***</u>

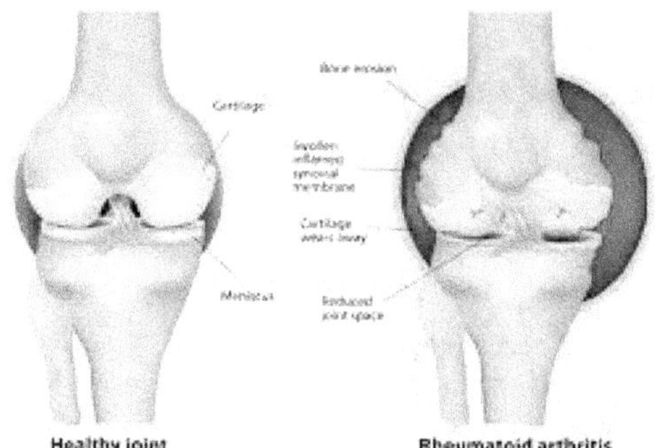

This is a condition that attacks the joints and causes swelling, pain, and loss of movement/mobility. There are dietary restrictions to help prevent the swelling:

• Avoid the nightshade vegetables like tomatoes, potatoes, eggplant, and peppers.

• Keeping a diary of what you eat and how your arthritis reacts to what you eat can add to that list of foods to avoid.

Eczema and Psoriasis

These are skin conditions that are visible on the skin and can range from rashes that are cracked and bleeding to scale-like rashes that weep. Even though there are prescription medications that claim to bring these conditions under control, but they do it by suppressing the immune system, which can expose you to more serious diseases.

There are two ways to start being proactive when it comes to controlling these conditions:

• Get an allergy test. It have been proven, in some cases, these are allergic reactions to either environmental factors or food you eat.

• Manage your stress. This is easier said than done, but learning how to relieve and control stress will work wonders for controlling and, in some cases, relieve the condition altogether.

Bruise Salve

1 Cup of Sweet Almond oil (or Apricot Kernel oil if you're allergic to tree nuts)
1/8 Cup Beeswax
1 Tbsp _Arnica flowers_
(Really good for bruises)
1 Tbsp _Lavender Flowers_
(Good for Swelling)
(You can substitute Chamomile here)
1 Tbsp _Echinacea_
(Speeds healing)

Bruise poultice

2 Tbsp Arnica Flowers
Echinacea Tea

Joint Muscle Rub

6 Ounces of Sweet Almond Oil
2 Ounces of Olive Oil
2 Tbsp Juniper Berries
(Swelling and joint pain)
2 Tbsp Devil's Claw
(Joint pain and ligaments)
1 Tbsp Cinnamon
(Swelling and heating effect)
2 Tbsp Peppermint Leaves
(Cooling effect and anti-inflammatory)

Joint Herbal Bath

1/2 Ounce of Juniper Berries
1/2 Ounce of Lavender or Chamomile Flowers

Eczema Ointment

2 Tbsp Kelp (Smooths the skin)
2 Tbsp Chamomile Flowers (helps smooth skin)
2 Tbsp Echinacea
2 Tbsp Avocado Butter (for extra moisture)

Psoriasis Rub

1/4 Cup Shea Butter
1/4 Cup Avocado Butter
(Both are excellent to toning and softening the skin and adding moisture)
2 Tbsp Lavender flowers
2 Tbsp Rose Petals
2 Tbsp Peppermint Leaves
1/4 ounce Aloe leaf

- Place the butters in a crock pot
- Add the herbs and steep overnight
- Strain out the herbs and place in a container with a tight lid.
- Let it cool before completely tightening the lid.
- Rub into the patches.

The Circulatory System

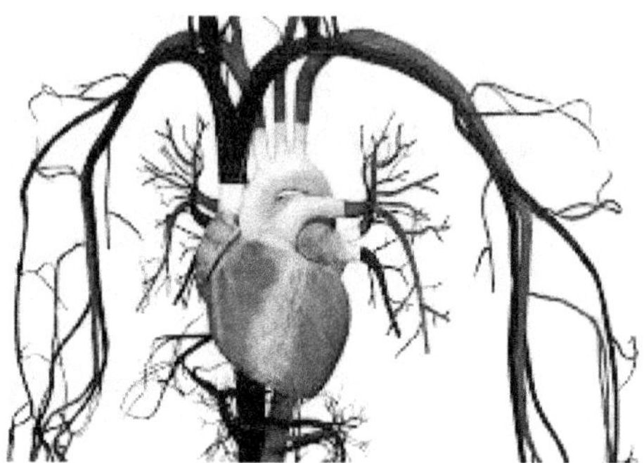

Your heart and blood vessels are the carriers of the oxygen that leaves you lungs. They also help you convey vitamins, minerals, and amino acids to your muscles. When your blood vessels start to clog, you can experience shortness of breath, low energy, and put your heart at risk because it's trying to work harder to get the blood to where it needs to go.

Heart disease and hypertension are two of the most prominent problems in our society. Taking care of your heart is very important for a healthy life.

Hypertension

Simply put this is very high blood pressure on a regular/daily basis. Left untreated, it can lead to heart attack and stroke.

As the skin condition above, relieving and learning how to manage stress can help lower blood pressure.

Changes in diet can do this as well. Even walking three times a week for at least twenty minutes can reduce your blood pressure. Here are a couple of recipes that can help without interacting with any medications you may be taking.

For a Weak Heart

Some people are born with congenital heart disease or a weak heart. This leads to them tiring easily and being short of breath.

Infusion for weak valves

1 tsp hawthorn berries crushed
(Highly recommended for a weak heart)
1 tsp night blooming cereus
(for valve malfunctions)
1 tsp catnip
(nervine)
Makes 1 therapeutic strength cup or 3 6-ounce regular strength cups.

Post-op Heart Attack Decoction

1 tsp hawthorn berries
1 tsp Dan Sheng Root
(Helps speed healing from heart operations)
1 tsp Lemon Zest (for flavor)
1 tsp Lavender flowers
(reduces swelling)

Hypertension

Just cooking with Basil and Cardamom can help to reduce your blood pressure. You can find these at any grocery store. Cooking with flaxseed is another way to help reduce your blood pressure.

Tea for Hypertension

Ginger tea is excellent for hypertension but if you can't handle the bite you can add Lavender and a little raw orange juice.

<u>***Blood Builders***</u>

These two recipes are to help strengthen blood vessels and for those who have low iron in their blood.

Iron Tea

1 tsp Red Raspberry leaves
1 tsp Red Clover flowers cut
1 tsp Butcher's Broom

Varicose Vein Bath

1/2 ounce Butcher's Broom
1/2 ounce Burdock Root

<u>*Migraines*</u>

There are headaches that can be a nuisance and there are migraines that can make chunks of your absolutely miserable with a spike is driven through your head. Thought they are still trying to figure out all the root causes of migraines there are few things you can do to help stave some of them off:

- Log smells, foods and other things that can trigger a migraine.
- High stress can also cause migraines.

You can help relieve stress by meditation, and listening to soothing music when you come home from a busy day.

Migraine Tea

1 tsp Feverfew
1 tsp Peppermint

The Glandular System

This is the system that can regulate everything from the metabolism to you hormones and everything in between. Even though the liver is generally considered part of the digestive system, I have put it here because of it's filtering abilities and how it aids the pancreas in regulating blood sugar levels.

Diabetes

This is a well-known disease which involves the pancreas. Insulin is created by the pancreas to regulate blood sugar, but when starts to malfunction, it can produce less and less, leading to higher levels of glucose in the blood.

This can cause dizziness and fainting spells, mood swings, and in more severe cases diabetic comas.

Nopal can help regulate glucose levels, and Stevia, a natural sweetener that is 10x sweeter than sugar, can as well.

Blood Sugar Tea

1 tsp Juniper Berries
1 tsp Ginger
1 tsp Billberry

Blood sugar Capsules

Equal parts of the following herbs in powder form:

Juniper berries

Nopal

Billberry

Stevia

It is recommended that you constantly check your blood sugar level if you are already on medication for this to make sure you are not lowering your glucose levels to dangerous numbers.

The Liver

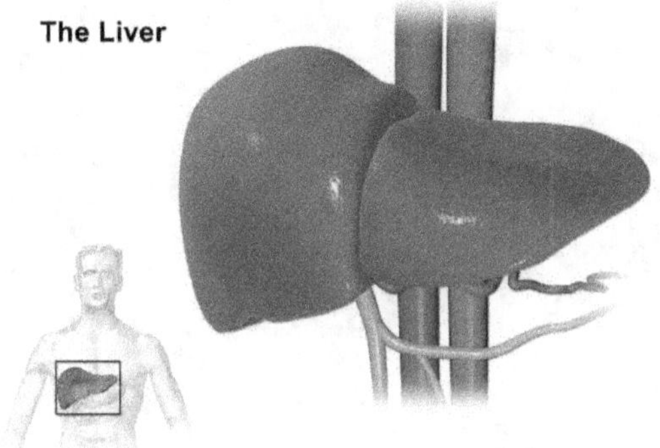

Your liver and gall bladder take the brunt of the abuse when it comes to filtering out any toxins in your system. From fats to alcohol and even artificial additives, these two glands work hard to make sure you will not get ill from toxicity, but when they are overworked, you can run into problems.

Detox Tea

1 tsp Milk thistle seeds
(excellent for detoxing the liver)
1 tsp Dandelion root
(good for liver and water retention)

<u>***Prostate***</u>

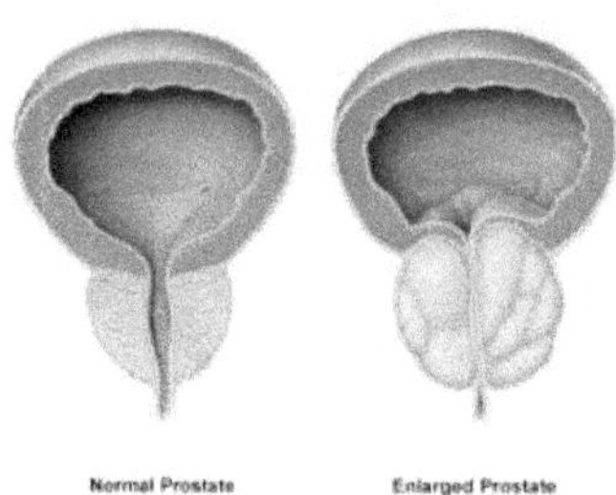

Prostate health is very important for men. Regular checks can lead to early detection for cancer and other prostate problems. There is also something you can take to maintain prostate health.

Saw Palmetto is the best supplement you take on a regular basis to maintain prostate health.

Conclusion

If someone you are with becomes seriously hurt you may need to assist them by moving them from location to location. Having that said, this means that you need to know the *proper way* to move them. If there are signs of a back injury for example, you need to make sure that the patient is rendered immobile in order to prevent any further injury to the back and neck. If you have someone to help you lift this person, that's great, but if you are by yourself you may just have to improvise.

One easy way to move someone would be to use a large article of clothing such as a bed sheet, or large coat to drag the individual. This is done by wrapping the clothing securely around the person's legs. You can then pull your ailing comrade to safety, it may not be the prettiest or most sophisticated way to render aid, but when all else fails, it will get the job done.

Administering CPR

Standing for "cardiopulmonary resuscitation", the technique called CPR is used to apply manual pressure to a heart that has stopped beating. In order to apply CPR, make sure the patient is on their back, on a flat surface. Now kneel beside the patient, positioning in line with their chest. Now place your index finger at the bottom notch of the person's ribs.

Position your hand's heel above this notch. Now place the palm of your hand on top of the other positioned above the notch. Now you can begin your chest compressions. Use a compression rate of 80 to 100 per minute, and stop every 15 to breathe 2 breaths into the person's lungs in between compressions. This emergency prep could be invaluable during a crisis.

Applying a Tourniquet

It's a gruesome reality, but if someone is injured severely enough, they can bleed to death. In order to prevent a tragedy like this, you need to know how to apply a tourniquet. Tourniquet's can be self-applied or applied to others, and simply consist of a material being wrapped around a limb in order to apply pressure and stem the flow of bleeding.

You can make a simple tourniquet simply by ripping a strip of cloth off of your shirt and tying it tightly around the affected area. Make sure the material is at least an inch and a half wide to make sure that it doesn't break and will remain stable. Keep this tourniquet on until you can stabilize the patient.

Giving Heimlich maneuver

If you see someone with a look of clear distress, with their face contorted in fear, unable to speak, unable to even breathe, and they are pointing to their throat, you can be sure that they are choking. In such a desperate situation the Heimlich maneuver is just what the survival doctor ordered. In order to properly administer this life saving maneuver, you need to stand directly behind the choking victim and place your arms around their stomach as if you are giving them a hug.

Now ball your hand into a fist and grab the outside of this fist with your other hand. Now with your elbows pointed out behind you begin energetically thrusting that fist up into the person's stomach causing the wind to shoot up through their diaphragm. This will eventually cause whatever is obstructing their windpipe to shoot out of their mouth. This bit of survival medicine really could save someone's life.